CBD: Cannabidiol

Legal Hemp for Health

Joanne Hillyer

ISBN:
9781520390802

CONTENTS

INTRODUCTION

Thank you for taking the time to download this book: *CBD: Cannabidiol —
Legal Hemp for Health.*

My passion is health and wellness, especially forms and methods that are
alternative to traditional/pharmaceutical medicine. This book covers the
topic of cannabidiol (abbreviated as CBD), and the history and use of the
medicinal hemp plant for health.

By the end of this book you will have a good understanding of what CBD
is, how it's different from the marijuana as a recreational drug, and its uses.

Once again, thank you for your purchase of this book, I hope you find it to
be helpful!

1 WHAT YOU NEED TO KNOW ABOUT MARIJUANA

This is a book that explains what the chemical component of marijuana called cannabidiol (CBD) is, and how it is used to improve one's health and treat various medical conditions.

To understand CBD, a discussion of the parent plant that is marijuana is first necessary. The properties that make CBD medicinal are inherent in marijuana. And so, we shall have in this first chapter a detailed look at marijuana or cannabis, the plant from which CBD is extracted.

The Hemp Plant and How It Is Grown

The marijuana plant is called *Cannabis sativa*, or more simply, hemp plant. Cannabis is the genus name, while the species is sativa. Two other Cannabis species exist, namely indica and ruderalis. It is *Cannabis sativa* that is the most widespread and well-known of the three. This specie is cultivated in many parts of the world for industrial hemp, and can be a source of medicinal and recreational marijuana as well. Meanwhile, *Cannabis indica* is primarily used to produce recreational and medicinal marijuana, and not grown for industrial hemp, because of its poor fiber quality. Apart from the three species, there are hybrids in between that are combinations of two or three of the original species.

Cannabis is an herb and a shrub. It has leaves, flowers, stems, and roots. It has palmate compound leaves, each leaf consisting of anywhere from 1 to

13 serrate leaflets. Leaves consisting of seven to nine leaflets are the most common. You may have seen drawings of the marijuana leaf in clothes or as logos, attesting — for better or worse — to the weed culture that is very popular worldwide, especially in hippie (and hip) communities.

When growing in the wild, the hemp plant has very long roots that are about as long as the part of the plant that is above ground. In other words, when you see wild *Cannabis sativa*, you are looking at half the plant, as the other half is hidden underground corresponding to the roots. In contrast, potted and indoor Cannabis (or those cultivated by people) has a much shorter root system. This is because the soil used by private or commercial growers is usually more nutrient-dense than the soil in the wild. Thus, the roots don't need to grow so long in order to get the water and sustenance they need.

When the leaves, flowers, and flower buds of the hemp plant are dried and shredded, the resulting grayish-green or brownish-green mixture is called marijuana. It is also referred to in slang by a variety of other names: pot, grass, weed, herb, ganja, MJ or Mary Jane, hash, reefer, sinsemilla, hemp, boom, gangster, dope, and so on.

Marijuana can be smoked or inhaled, drank like tea, or eaten as when mixed in with brownies, cookies, and other food. It has an intoxicating effect, producing a high that can be addictive. It is classified as a controlled substance, and its recreational use isn't legal in many states. Possession and cultivation of the plant are also felonies in those states, as is distribution of the drug.

Other parts of the Cannabis plant serve a more practical purpose. The stems and roots are primarily used to make hemp fiber and oil, and are known as "industrial hemp." These don't produce an inebriating effect because, firstly, they aren't taken into the body like the parts of the marijuana plant are for use as a drug, and secondly, they don't contain the hallucinogenic chemicals found in great concentrations in the flowers and leaves of the plant. Hemp fiber is used to make fabrics (such as canvas), rope, paper, textiles, and fuel oil (often as lamp oil). Hempseed and hemp oil are also useful as food and dietary supplements. We will discuss more about these uses in the coming chapters.

The hemp plant thrives best in humid and tropical places, but it can grow in most climates. It is, in fact, possible to grow anywhere in the world, because it can be cultivated indoors in a controlled environment. In fact, many growers prefer to plant it indoors or in private yards to avoid detection, because it is, after all, illegal to cultivate in many parts of the world including many states in the United States.

Without any legal restriction, Cannabis would be a grower's ideal plant. It is easy to take care of, it grows fast, and it is naturally resistant to many plant diseases. It also requires very little weeding. It is even known to enrich the soil it is planted in.

The Origins and Early History of Cannabis

Cannabis sativa is believed to have originated in central Asia in the Himalayan region. The enduring herb has been around for a long time. Archeological finds indicate that even in prehistoric times, Cannabis was already being used for its psychoactive (mind-altering) properties. In Africa and Euro-Asia, early people probably used Cannabis as a relaxant and pain reliever.

Among the earliest evidence of marijuana use are burned cannabis seeds excavated in burial mounds in Siberia. These have been dated to as far back as 3000 B.C. — more than four thousand years ago. Similarly, large amounts of mummified marijuana was also found in the tombs of aristocrats in the Xinjiang area in China, dating all the way to 2500 B.C.

From China, the use of marijuana spread to neighboring Korea in circa 2000 B.C., and then on to the South Asian region, particularly in India, between 2000 to 1000 B.C.

In written history, the earliest mention of the use of Cannabis in the Western world was in circa 440 B.C. The famous Greek historian Herodotus wrote about the Scythians of central Eurasia taking Cannabis steam baths and deriving great pleasure from those. Obviously, this is a reference to the recreational use of the plant. The Greeks and Romans also used marijuana and hemp, for both recreational and utilitarian purposes, as did the Muslims in North Africa. (It is worth noting that the Arabic word "hashish" or "hash," referring to smoked marijuana and literally meaning "dry weed," has been adopted as an English word.) With the spread of the Islamic Empire, Cannabis use expanded to the western hemisphere, mainly through the wide-ranging explorations of the Spaniards in various parts of the world. By the 1500s, Cannabis was already extensively grown in both North and South America.

Uses of Cannabis

A lot of people mistake Cannabis or marijuana for being just a recreational drug and nothing more. This cannot be further from the truth. While the leaves and flowers of the hemp plant are indeed used to produce pot, these and its other parts — the stems, roots, and seeds — are also made into hemp fiber, rope, paper, building materials and textiles.

Another byproduct of the plant is hemp oil, which can be consumed as food, used as fuel, or made into an ingredient in lotions, cosmetics, and other body care products. Lastly, and of perhaps the greatest value, the hemp plant serves medicinal purposes.

As food products, hempseed and hemp oil are nutritious and delicious. They too are excellent sources of protein, dietary fiber, fatty acids, and minerals. Hemp has in fact been singled out as the only plant that contains all of the essential amino acids and fatty acids needed by the human body. Hemp also is the preferred option for many vegetarians who are averse to taking fish and fish oil supplements.

As textile and fabric, hemp products are similar to cotton but are more durable. Many rugs, ropes, nets, sails, and ship riggings are made from hemp. Canvas is another durable byproduct of hemp (the Latin origin of the word canvas literally means hemp). Interestingly, the original Levi Strauss' denim jeans and the first American flag were made from hemp.

As a fuel, hemp oil was traditionally used to light lamps. It had been used as such for many centuries, until petroleum largely replaced it in the late 1800s. At present, hemp oil is utilized more as a biofuel to replace gasoline for car engines. It is a renewable and environment-friendly alternative to fossil fuels.

As building materials, hemp products are used much like wood to construct homes and structures. They are used to make walls, panels, pipes, foundations, shingles, and even paint. Modern hemp building materials have been reinvented to make them fireproof, waterproof, and pest-resistant, apart from being lightweight.

As an illicit drug, marijuana is often smoked in hand-rolled cigarettes — nicknamed "joints" — or with the use of bongs or pipes. It can also be smoked in the form of blunts — marijuana cigars made by cutting regular cigars open and replacing the tobacco inside with weed. Marijuana can also be consumed by mouth, as when it is mixed with common food such as cookies, candies, and brownies. Other forms of marijuana are the so-called "hash oil," which has the appearance of honey; "shatter," which looks like hard amber, and the waxy "budder." These are concentrated concoctions with high doses of marijuana. These have recently become the preferred drugs of both recreational and medical users of marijuana.

Over the years, many strains of Cannabis have been developed and bred to suit any of the specific purposes discussed above. Some Cannabis strains produce abundant fiber. These are ideal for use in making industrial hemp products. Other strains have been bred to contain very low amounts of the psychoactive chemical component known as tetrahydrocannabinol (THC) so as to remove the hallucinogenic effect when taking Cannabis. This then makes their use "safe" enough for medicinal applications and compliant to narcotics laws. Yet other strains have been developed to produce very high levels of THC, catering to the desires of recreational drug users. These strains often fetch high prices in the black market. Up to the present time, there is a massive, ongoing research and development on Cannabis and its various uses and applications.

Marijuana as a Medicinal Drug

The general perception of marijuana is overwhelmingly negative, as it is well known for being a psychedelic drug. In recent decades, a shift in perception has occurred, and now, more and more people are becoming aware of the medicinal benefits of the hemp plant.

The fact is that marijuana has been used for medicinal purposes for thousands of years already. Medicinal marijuana was used in ancient China, and then in other parts of Asia and on to the Middle East and the African continent. Its main medicinal use was as an anesthetic or pain reliever. While it was used for this purpose, traditional medicine at the same time cautioned against abusing the plant or using too much of it. Doctors warned their patients that excessive marijuana use could lead to hallucinations or "seeing demons."

Marijuana also was used to treat a wide range of ailments in ancient China. These conditions ranged from poor memory to malaria, sleeplessness to gout, and anorexia (loss of appetite) to rheumatism. No less than the Chinese emperor Shen Neng in 2737 B.C. officially prescribed marijuana as a cure for those particular ailments.

Apart from the Chinese, the Indians and Hindus also embraced the use of marijuana for both recreational and medicinal purposes, and even for religious and spiritual uses. As early as the year 2000 B.C., special drinks and concoctions of Cannabis were part of Indian culture. An example is the drink called *bhang*, which is made of milk, spices, ghee, and Cannabis paste (taken from Cannabis leaves and flower buds). Specific mention of bhang can be seen in the Indian scripture called the Vedas. The fourth Vedic book refers to bhang as an herb mixture that releases a person from anxiety. Later writings and records also lauded bhang for its ability to "remove wind and phlegm," improve mental ability, and make one feel warm and happy.

There are countless similar accounts in the ancient world of the use of marijuana as medicine (and as a psychoactive substance). These accounts make for an interesting and highly informative read. We shall look at this fascinating history of the plant throughout the ages and in different parts of the world in a later chapter.

Marijuana as a Controlled Substance

Of all prohibited drugs, Cannabis is the most commonly used worldwide. Statistics reveal that in 2014, close to 185 million people globally were marijuana users, and the majority of these were teenagers. One reason for the widespread use of Cannabis may be that it is relatively easy to acquire. It is also not difficult to grow by oneself. Anyone can easily search on the Internet for how-to guides on growing marijuana and find many answers.

Another reason for its popularity is the perception that marijuana is much less harmful than the truly "hardcore" drugs such as cocaine or methamphetamines. Many people think of marijuana as an herb that is natural and organic (versus being synthetic), hence it cannot really be bad for anyone. In their mind, using weed can't be much more damaging than eating any other herb or vegetable.

The reality, however, is that marijuana is a controlled substance with many potentially destructive effects on the user's health and behavior. Studies have established that marijuana use weakens neurological functions. It impairs short-term memory, learning, mental focus, and motor coordination. It causes hallucinations. Among young users, there also is evidence of declining IQ levels when they reach adulthood. Using weed also can lead to abnormally high heart rates and palpitations, and lung damage (when smoked). It further increases the risk of psychosis among vulnerable people, specifically those with a history of or susceptibility towards mental illness. Pregnant women and breastfeeding mothers who use marijuana further run the risk of having low-birth-weight babies with possible cognitive underdevelopment.

While this has not been wholly proven, many people believe that marijuana is addictive. Among adult users, one out of every nine (or roughly 9 percent) develops a dependency on the drug. The risk for addiction increases when regular use begins in the adolescent years; in this case, one person out of every six users (17 percent) runs the risk for dependency.

In summary, below are the negative effects of marijuana use.

Short-term effects of using marijuana:

- Forgetfulness and memory problems

- Severe anxiety, which can develop into paranoia (the irrational fear of being watched or followed)

- Hallucinations, or seeing, hearing, or smelling things that aren't really there

- Psychosis, or the inability to distinguish between reality and imagination or hallucinations

- Strange behavior resulting from psychosis and hallucinations

- Panic and anxiety

- No sense of personal identity

- Coordination problems and decreased reaction time, making it dangerous when playing sports, driving or operating machinery

- Very high heart rates that could lead to heart palpitations

- Greater risk for stroke and heart attack

- Sexual problems (for males)

- Much greater risk among females for contracting sexually transmitted diseases (STDs) than non-users

Long-term effects of marijuana use:

- A decrease in IQ of up to 8 points if regular drug use started in the teenage years

- Poor performance in school or at work

- Higher chance of dropping out of school

- Greater chance of being unemployed, not landing good jobs, and the inability to stay employed for long

- Impaired thinking, and difficulty in learning and doing complex tasks

- A general dissatisfaction with life that can develop into depression

- Addiction to marijuana

- Possible development of greater opiate abuse. Marijuana has been described as a "gateway" drug, which means that it leads to further experimentation and use of other, more harmful drugs.

- Relationship and social problems, including domestic violence

- Antisocial and criminal activities, including lying and stealing

- Financial difficulties

Ordinarily, not all nor even many of these effects will be experienced by marijuana users. In fact, the majority of users experience very little of these negative effects; what they get is mostly just the high, relaxation, or inebriation they were after. If a recreational user smokes marijuana only occasionally and in small amounts, he probably won't suffer any serious health impairment. But every person reacts differently to the drug. Some are more sensitive to it than others.

2 Common Myths About Marijuana

There is a lot of information out there about marijuana, and this is good because being knowledgeable helps a person make better choices. Someone trying to decide whether to use medical marijuana or not should certainly get all the facts straight.

The trouble is that we simply can't take everything we read or hear about as 100 percent accurate. One must do some research on his own and learn to discriminate which pieces of information are reliable and which aren't. We should be aware that big stakes are involved in the marijuana debate. Large corporations and powerful groups are concerned about how the public perceives marijuana — that is, if it should be legalized or not, and if the benefits it brings outweigh the bad effects. As such, these groups could be manipulating the type of information that comes out in the open, to lead to outcomes that are favorable to their interests but are not necessarily aligned with the general public's.

Another thing to consider is that science cannot and does not always give definite answers to some questions. Scientific studies, especially in the early stages of research and development, can produce conflicting findings and conclusions. New evidence can at any time surface to disprove what was previously thought of as factual.

What is clear is that there has been a strong and long-standing stigma against marijuana. Those who are opposed to its use have long controlled the messaging concerning this valuable but misunderstood plant. Now, slowly, this stigma is weakening, and there is greater acceptance of the possibility that marijuana could be more helpful than harmful. That it has been legalized in many American states is solid proof of this acceptance.

With these in mind, let us look at some long-established views about marijuana that most people take as truth, yet may not be very factual at all. Proponents of marijuana call these misconceptions and myths that must be debunked so that we all can correctly appreciate what marijuana is, what it isn't, and what it can or can't do.

Myth #1: Driving with a marijuana high is as bad as drunk driving

There is no evidence that being stoned while driving causes as many road accidents as drunk driving does. It is even being debated whether stoned driving actually increases the incidence of traffic accidents. While the disastrous effects of drunk driving have been amply supported by evidence — approximately 28 people every day are killed because of drunk driving — no such numbers exist for stoned driving.

It is true that being high on weed does impair motor function and slow down reaction time. However, marijuana proponents argue that knowing this makes users so much more cautious. After using, they then decide not to drive at all, or to be very vigilant and careful when they do decide to drive. As a result, they don't cause as many road accidents as drunk drivers do.

Furthermore, there is evidence indicating that while high, regular pot smokers experience less impairment when driving compared to occasional users. This could mean that over time, marijuana smokers gain enough control over their stoned state to enable them to drive safely.

Myth #2: Marijuana use leads to brain damage

The effects of using weed on the brain are more short-lived than long-term. Smoking weed causes short-term memory problems, anxiety, hallucinations, coordination, and motor problems. The long-term effects aren't as well established; they are presented as possible or probable effects that may or may not actually happen. These long-term effects include poor performance in school or at work, a greater chance of not finishing school or getting a stable job, addiction, and lowered IQ. The last item in the list — a lowered IQ — may sound suggestive of serious mental deterioration, but it warrants further scrutiny. A decrease in IQ for people who started using early in life isn't an established certainty. There are no statistics to positively confirm this, but there are indeed indications that it does happen to some people.

The fact remains that marijuana use has not been proven to alter brain functioning permanently, nor has it been proven to cause brain damage. It also does not kill brain cells. There had been isolated research findings suggesting that marijuana use "reorganizes" the brain or changes its structure, but these were later cleared up as misreported or misinterpreted conclusions by the press.

Myth #3: Smoking weed destroys the lungs the way smoking cigarettes does

Is smoking weed worse for the lungs than smoking cigarettes? There is no clear scientific evidence of this. On the other hand, what many research findings support is the observation that occasional or non-habitual use of marijuana does not negatively affect the body's respiratory or pulmonary function, instead long-term regular use will result in pulmonary problems because smoke is an irritant to lung tissue. However, this isn't to say that the damage will be worse than that caused by smoking cigarettes.

Comparing cigarette and weed smokers, there is a significant difference in the quantities each group smokes. Heavy cigarette smokers are known to consume one to two packs a day, while heavy pot smokers don't usually go beyond three or four joints or bowls in a day. As a result, cigarette smokers cause significantly greater damage to their lungs, simply because they smoke much, much more than the amount weed smokers do. Thus, marijuana users tend to have healthier lungs and better pulmonary function than cigarette smokers.

Another thing to bear in mind is that smoking isn't the only way of taking marijuana. Users can ingest cannabis in many ways that don't expose their lungs to noxious smoke. They can eat marijuana, drink it, vaporize and inhale it without smoke, or take it in tablet form. With these methods, the lungs will suffer no damage.

Myth #4: Legalization of marijuana would benefit drug cartels

If marijuana were 100 percent legalized, this would weaken drug cartels. These cartels make money not just from actually producing or distributing marijuana, but also through extortion, human trafficking, and other various criminal activities. With the legalization (or de-criminalization) of the drug, these activities would cease considerably. There would not be much need for criminal drug organizations to extort from people, bribe government officials and politicians, or train and arm their soldiers.

The fact is that drug cartels are more active in countries and regions where drug use is illegal. They do not normally operate in places where the drug has been legalized.

Myth #5: Legalization will encourage greater recreational use of pot, especially among the youth

The year 2011 saw the highest incidence of marijuana use among teenagers in the United States. Statistics showed that close to 7 percent of all high school students — the highest figure recorded in 30 years — smoked pot almost daily. This number even exceeded the number of teenagers who smoked cigarettes.

The point is that the use of marijuana can increase among young people even without the legalization of the drug. In other words, it isn't legalizing weed (or medical marijuana) that results in a higher incidence of its use.

Furthermore, there are no statistics to prove that there is a higher number of adolescent pot smokers in states where marijuana is legal compared to those in other states where it isn't legal. This means that teens do not smoke any more pot in states where marijuana is legal.

Advocates for the legalization of marijuana argue that this move could in fact protect young people because marijuana use would then be regulated.

Myth #6: A person can overdose on weed and die

Experts have determined that the lethal dose of weed, meaning the dose that can kill a person, is close to 40,000 times the regular dose. Thus, if the regular dose for a person is, say, three joints, then he needs to smoke something like 120,000 joints in one sitting to die from marijuana overdose. This just doesn't happen because it is physically impossible.

3 A SHORT HISTORY OF THE USE OF MARIJUANA

Let us examine some selected historical highlights that outline the spread and use of the plant. In this fascinating list, we don't just get to know about notable incidents in the long chronology of marijuana, but we also see how people used weed for various therapeutic applications. Also of interest is the involvement of a few important persons in the history of the drug.

- The earliest written reference to medical Cannabis is in 1500 B.C. in the Chinese Pharmacopeia called Rh-Ya.

- In 1450 B.C., mention is made in the Book of Exodus of a "holy anointing oil" made of kaneh-bosem (a local name for Cannabis), olive oil, and some aromatic herbs. This is among the earliest references to the use of marijuana for spiritual and religious ceremonies.

- In 1213 B.C., Egyptian healers used Cannabis to cure inflammation, glaucoma and abdominal problems. Cannabis was also used when administering enemas.

- In 1000 B.C., Indians drank *bhang*, a concoction of Cannabis and milk, and used this recreationally and as a medical anesthetic.

- In 600 B.C., marijuana is cited in Indian medical literature as a cure for leprosy. In the treatise Sushruta Samhita, Cannabis is further cited as a tonic that prolongs life, improves thinking and judgment, cures fevers, improves the quality of sleep, and cures dysentery.

- In 200 B.C., Greeks used marijuana to cure edema (swelling), earache, and inflammation.

- In 1 A.D., a Chinese text commended marijuana as a helpful remedy for no fewer than a hundred ailments. It further claimed that the drug is most effective in treating gout, rheumatism, and malaria, and in improving memory.

- In 30 A.D., Jesus is believed to have used cannabis oil when anointing his followers.

- In 70 A.D., marijuana was used by Roman doctors medicinally to cure earache and "suppress sexual longing."

- In 200 A.D., Chinese doctors used *ma-yo*, an anesthetic agent made from marijuana and wine, when performing surgical operations.

- In 800 A.D., some Arabic doctors lauded the effectiveness of marijuana as an anesthetic and an analgesic (pain reliever), while others cautioned using it because it is a "lethal poison."

- In 1578, the medical treatise by Li Shizhen, titled *Bencao Gangmu Materia Medica*, cites marijuana as a potent cure for vomiting, hemorrhage (bleeding), and parasitic infections. At the same time, the drug was a popular folk remedy for dysentery and diarrhea, and as an appetite stimulant.

- In the 1600s, the famous English poet William Shakespeare may have smoked marijuana. A number of pipes, bowls, and stems allegedly belonging to him were recovered and forensically examined. Some of these contained vestiges of tobacco, marijuana, and even cocaine. It is believed that like many other artists and creative people, Shakespeare enjoyed Cannabis as a stimulant that helped spark greater creativity.

- Between 1611 and 1762, the first settlers in Jamestown introduced Cannabis to North America. They brought with them the hemp plant and cultivated it for its fiber and oil, and for recreational/medical use. It is worth noting that in Virginia in 1762, bounties were awarded for hemp cultivation and manufacture, and penalties were imposed on planters who failed to produce it.

- In 1621, a popular English book called *The Anatomy of Melancholy* came into print; it recommended marijuana as a cure for depression.

- In 1625, the renowned and influential English herbalist Nicholas Culpeper wrote of the many uses of hemp extract. He lauded it as a remedy for gout pain, head inflammations, and muscular and joint pain. This is probably one of the earliest medical applications of non-psychoactive (low-THC) marijuana.

- Between 1745 and 1775, the future U.S. president George Washington grew hemp in his plantation at Mount Vernon. He cultivated Cannabis that had high THC content. He was deeply interested in the medicinal uses of the plant, and probably used it recreationally too, as his diaries reveal.

- Between 1774 and 1824, in Monticello, Virginia, another U.S. president, Thomas Jefferson, also grew hemp. But unlike George Washington, there is no evidence that Jefferson smoked hemp or even tobacco as a habit.

- In the late 1700s, the French emperor Napoleon invaded Egypt and brought to the country a scientific expedition team. This team not only discovered the Rosetta Stone, but also brought Cannabis back with them when they returned to France in 1799. They studied and developed the plant for its sedative and analgesic properties. This helped introduce marijuana in mainstream Western medicine.

- In 1842 or thereabouts, the famous Irish doctor William O-Shaughnessy reintroduced marijuana into British medicine when he got back from his stint as an army surgeon in British-controlled India. Cannabis became very popular in Britain, with reports alleging that Queen Victoria herself used it as pain reliever when she had menstrual cramps. Her personal physician, Sir Robert Russell, wrote comprehensively about marijuana, citing it as a very effective treatment for dysmenorrhea (menstrual pain). Other uses for Cannabis in the Victorian era were for rheumatism, insomnia, muscle spasms, convulsions related to tetanus, epilepsy, rabies, and to stimulate uterine contractions in childbirth. At this time, medical Cannabis was used in the form of tincture that was taken orally, rather than smoked.

- By the 1840s, marijuana had become part of mainstream medicine in Europe. Apart from the English, the French also used Cannabis commonly as a pain reliever and as medicine to treat sleeplessness and loss of appetite.

- By the 1850s, medicinal Cannabis had also gone mainstream in the United States. It was catalogued in the United States Pharmacopeia (the official inventory of prescription and over-the-counter medicines) as a cure for a long list of ailments. The medical conditions that marijuana was used for included alcoholism, rabies, cholera, abnormal menstrual and uterine bleeding, gout, convulsions, leprosy, typhus, tetanus, anthrax, neuralgia (nerve pain), tonsillitis, insanity, opiate addiction, incontinence, dysentery, and many others. The tincture form of Cannabis was the standard therapeutic method used.

- In 1889, leading medical journals emphasized the effectiveness of Cannabis in relieving withdrawal symptoms related to opium use. Cannabis helped reduce cravings for opium and relieved nausea and vomiting among patients undergoing rehab for substance addiction.

- From 1893 to 1900 in India and South Asia, official medical journals recognized the efficacy of Cannabis treatment for a variety of conditions including but not limited to the following asthma, cholera, bronchitis, chronic ulcers, gonorrhea, diabetes, sexual dysfunction, hay fever, loss of appetite, dysentery, and urinary incontinence. The same official publications also reported that medical Cannabis was used in both rural areas and in the urban centers. In this same time period, a commission in India was formed to look into the increasingly widespread use of marijuana as an intoxicant and a recreational drug.

- In 1911, Massachusetts became the first state in the U.S. to officially declare Cannabis as a dangerous drug and ban its use. This occurred simultaneously with a crackdown on crimes and vices such as prostitution, gambling, prizefighting, and alcohol abuse.

- From 1913 to 1917, other states followed the example of Massachusetts and declared Cannabis use as illegal. These states included Maine, Indiana, Wyoming, New York City, Utah, Vermont, Colorado, and Nevada. Cannabis use wasn't really a major problem at that time, but there was a proliferation of vices that the government wished to eradicate. Cannabis got caught in the tide of reforms during these so-called "prohibitionist years" that attempted to reduce crime and to restore high moral values among the people.

What followed afterwards was mostly the passing and implementation of stricter laws against the use of marijuana. This was the trend not just in the U.S. but in many other countries. The U.K. and even international multi-country organizations declared Cannabis as a dangerous substance and in many cases imposed that its use be strictly for medical and scientific purposes only.

Ironically, marijuana use and production did not abate. In fact, it grew more widespread over the decades that followed.

In recent years, the trend has been towards the decriminalization and legalization of Cannabis as it has become evident that it is a very effective medicine and not nearly as dangerous or harmful to people's health as previously thought.

4 THE MAJOR CANNABINOIDS AND WHAT THEY DO

The active chemical components of Cannabis are called *cannabinoids*. There are no fewer than 85 types of cannabinoids in the hemp plant, and hundreds of other plant chemicals such as chlorophyll and lipids. We are interested in the cannabinoids because they are the ones that have been tested in laboratories and shown to possess the medicinal properties that marijuana has. Many of these cannabinoids also have psychoactive or hallucinogenic properties, meaning that they could get a person "high."

Cannabinoids have such a potent effect on the human body both medicinally and psychoactively because they work very much like the natural hormones already present in our body. These naturally occurring hormones are called *endogenous cannabinoids* or *endocannabinoids*. They fulfill a useful role in keeping the body healthy; they help maintain internal stability and facilitate communication between cells, in the same manner that brain neurotransmitters function. Endocannabinoids in fact work mostly as part of the nervous system. They affect areas in the brain that control memory, pleasure, cognition, coordination, movement, concentration, and the perception of time and space. These are exactly the same areas of the brain that are affected when a person uses marijuana.

The two most potent cannabinoids from marijuana are *cannabinoil* (CBD) and *delta-9-tetrahydrocannabinol* (THC). These two are the most highly studied because they are the major components of Cannabis. In other words, they are the two cannabinoids that have the highest concentrations compared to the other 80 or so active chemical components of the plant.

CBD has great medicinal value and no mind-altering properties. THC is less benign in that it is also highly medicinal *and* highly psychoactive. As such, THC has been nicknamed "the high causer," as it causes a person to feel high and intoxicated. Cannabis strains bred for recreational use contain higher amounts of THC compared to CBD. On the other hand, Cannabis strains cultivated for industrial purposes (to produce hemp fiber and oil) contain very little THC — too little to cause any psychological effects. Industrial Cannabis typically contains less than 0.3 percent THC, while recreational Cannabis strains usually have 6 percent to as much as 20 percent (or even higher) concentrations of THC.

When marijuana is smoked, CBD, THC, and other cannabinoids enter the bloodstream via the lungs. They then mimic the action of endocannabinoids and immediately bind to receptors in neurons in our brain. One positive effect this can have is to instantaneously provide relief from pain, nausea, and other symptoms of inflammation. On the negative side, another effect is to alter normal brain function. For example, it can cause forgetfulness, impaired thinking, lack of mental focus, and the proper sense of time and place. Medically speaking, these are unwanted side effects that should be avoided. Obviously, in normal living, they are unwanted effects as well because they negatively impact a person's health, his daily activities, social relationships, and work performance.

Cannabidiol (CBD): The Good Stuff?

Two things about CBD have already been mentioned in the preceding section. First, it is a chief chemical component of marijuana. Second, it doesn't have any psychoactive or mind-altering effects, meaning that it doesn't cause a high. This is considered to be a major advantage for proponents of medicinal marijuana because treatments and drugs that have the least number of side effects are naturally preferred. Medicines that don't have mind-altering properties are of course considered safer than those that impair mental processes.

Another advantage of CBD is its potency and versatility as a medicinal agent. Listed here are the various medical properties of CBD that have been documented in many research studies:

- CBD is an anti-inflammatory agent that helps reduce pain, swelling, fever and other symptoms of tissue or organ inflammation.

- It is antiemetic, meaning that it has the ability to lessen nausea and vomiting.

- It is also an anticonvulsant, therefore helpful in reducing and preventing seizures.

- It has antioxidant properties, helping to cure or reverse neurodegenerative ailments and delay the effects of aging.

- CBD has been used as an antipsychotic agent that helps improve mental health. It is also useful in reducing anxiety and depression.

- It is known to help destroy tumor and cancer cells.

Yet another good thing about CBD is that it reduces the psychoactive effects of THC. As mentioned, THC is undesirable in that it causes inebriation and mental impairment; it is what causes a person to feel stoned. When combined with CBD, this effect of THC is reduced. As shown in clinical tests, CBD gives a natural protection against the high and psychedelic effects of marijuana. As such, scientists sometimes refer to CBD as a "negative modulator" for THC.

With regard to its therapeutic uses, CBD has been found to be helpful in the treatment of a number of conditions, including diabetes, epilepsy in children and other related pediatric conditions, cancer, lupus and other auto-immune disorders, Parkinson's disease, osteoporosis, motor disorders, neuropathic pain, obsessive-compulsive (OCD) disorder, and addiction to nicotine. Overall, the greatest medicinal success of CBD has been in its effectiveness as a cure for epilepsy, anxiety, depression, and psychotic disorders.

THC: "The High Causer" and Therefore the Bad Guy?

The information provided so far seems to indicate that if a person wants to get high, he should go for marijuana strains that have high THC content, and conversely, if he wants medical relief without getting stoned, he should go for strains that have a high CBD and low THC content. This is some truth to this generalization, but it does not tell the whole story. THC is indeed the psychoactive component in marijuana, and is therefore "the bad guy" or the undesirable ingredient, but it does have some redeeming qualities as well. Let us look at some facts about THC below to clarify what we mean.

- While tetrahydrocannabinol or THC is the primary chemical in marijuana that makes a person high, it also has great medicinal value. It is known to relieve nausea and pain, cure depression and epilepsy, protect brain cells, stimulate greater mental activity, and provide many other medicinal benefits. There are in fact FDA-approved drugs that have THC as the main active ingredient. These include Dronabinol, a drug that relieves nausea and vomiting especially among patients going through chemotherapy.

- THC has been classified as a "neuroprotectant" — a chemical that protects brain cells from damage caused by normal age-related wear and tear and by inflammation. Furthermore, THC is also a "neurogenetic" agent, meaning a chemical that helps promote the growth of new brain cells and the regeneration of brain matter.

- Certain naturally occurring chemicals in the body are very closely similar in composition and action to THC. These chemicals, such as anandamide, are helpful to the body in that they help to regulate sleep, mood, appetite, and memory. There is every indication that THC can and does perform these same beneficial effects on the nervous system.

- THC doesn't always cause feelings of inebriation or euphoria. There is a "latent" form of THC that is called *tetrahydrocannabinolic acid* or THCA. This is the form that is present in Cannabis preparations that have not been exposed to heat or that are raw (uncooked). THCA is not psychoactive and will not make a person feel stoned. However, it converts into THC when exposed to heat through a process called decarboxylation. Here lies the reason why recreational users of weed do not want to eat it raw or use it without heating it in some way first: THCA won't give them the high they want, and so it must be converted to THC first before ingestion.

The Optimum CBD-THC Combination in Medicinal Marijuana

Many proponents of medicinal marijuana favor the use of Cannabis strains that have a high CBD content and zero-to-minimal amounts of THC. These are the so-called "CBD-dominant" strains, which do not produce any psychoactive effects when used. These are the Cannabis varieties that recreational users do not want.

Not everyone agrees that this is the CBD-THC combination that will bring about the greatest medicinal benefit. Research findings reveal that the therapeutic value of marijuana is maximized when combining the potency of both CBD and THC. This combination is more effective than CBD acting alone, or THC acting solely. Thus, some medical practitioners prefer the so-called "CBD-rich" strains instead of the CBD-dominant ones. These CBD-rich varieties are those that either have equal amounts of CBD and THC, or more CBD than THC.

Some examples of CBD-rich strains of marijuana are the Sour Tsunami, Harlequin, Omrita Rx, and Jamaican Lion. These have a CBD-to-THC ratio of about 3-to-2.

An example of a CBD-dominant strain goes by the colorful name of Women's Collective Stinky Purple. This contains about ten times more CBD than THC. Other strains of this type are Charlotte's Web, ACDC, Valentine X, and Cannatonic.

Distinguishing Among CBD and THC Oils, Cannabis Oil, Marijuana Oil and Other Variants

The terminologies involving CBD and various marijuana extracts and oils can be confusing, and so in this section we will clarify what these are and how they differ, if they aren't the same thing.

CBD oil, hemp oil, and Cannabidiol (CBD) are practically interchangeable terms. They refer to oil or extracts that contains mostly CBD and no THC. If they do have THC, it is in a very small and negligible concentration that is usually less than 0.3 percent of the total weight. These oils and products are legal to use in the United States, in Europe and in many parts of the world. They can easily be bought commercially. Numerous websites sell CBD oil online.

Meanwhile, Cannabis oil, also known as marijuana oil, can refer to either CBD oil or THC oil. The amounts of CBD and THC in it vary widely. Some Cannabis oil have a higher CBD content than THC, others have about equal amounts of CBD and THC, while still others have more THC than CBD. CBD-dominant marijuana oil is legal everywhere, while THC-dominant Cannabis oil isn't.

THC oil is Cannabis oil that obviously has a high THC content. It isn't legal country-wide (but it is in some states) because it can cause the user to experience a high. It is intended mostly for recreational use, but it has been known to possess medicinal properties too.

THC oil and high-THC marijuana oil (which are virtually the same) often contain extracts from imported Dutch marijuana oil. It is made by first extracting, with alcohol, the resin of the female Cannabis plant. The resin is then dissolved in alcohol, and alcohol is allowed to evaporate. The result is a thick syrup rich in THC. It may be mixed with or dissolved in hempseed oil so that it can be ingested orally more easily. In states where it isn't legal it is difficult to buy THC oil from commercial sources, but people have been known to make their own using instructions that can be gathered online.

Rick Simpson oil (RSO) is an example of THC oil. Its inventor, Rick Simpson, is a pioneer and activist for legalizing marijuana who claims to have cured his own cancer with RSO. He shares his methods of preparing RSO on his website and in books he has written.

Hemp oil, which we mentioned earlier as synonymous with CBD oil, can also refer to hempseed oil. Hempseed oil is edible, delicious, and rich in unsaturated fats, namely Omega 3 and Omega 6. It can be a dietary supplement. Hempseed oil usually does not contain either TCH or CBD because the seeds of the hemp plant do not have great amounts of either cannabinoid.

It is worth mentioning that some variants of CBD oil can contain other cannabinoids that are very similar to CBD but aren't exactly the same.

Examples of these chemicals are CBDA, CBC, CBGA, and CBCA. Their effects on the body when ingested or used as medicine approximate the effects of CBD, but are less potent. Sometimes, CBD oils with these CBD-like chemicals are mixed with hempseed oil or olive oil to produce an enhanced taste or better dosage.

5 MARIJUANA AS MEDICINE

In this chapter, we get to the nitty-gritty part and explore how marijuana can be used as medicine. We will look at the various methods of using medical Cannabis, the pros and cons of each, and some possible side effects from their use.

What Type of Cannabis Therapy Is Best for You?

A common question is, how does a person know if medical marijuana is for him? Which medical conditions warrant the use of medical Cannabis?

For many people, the answer is simple: If you are having trouble with pain, and you have tried the more conventional analgesic therapies but didn't get the relief that you wanted, then medical marijuana can very probably help you. It doesn't matter much what caused the pain, because marijuana can bring relief for anything from headaches to nerve pain. It is helpful for acute pain as well as for chronic pain resulting from long-term conditions such as glaucoma or cancer.

Additionally, to help you decide whether to use marijuana or not, it can be useful to consider the most common ailments for which Cannabis is prescribed by doctors. If your medical condition is one of them, then you will likely benefit from Cannabis therapy. Treatment with cannabinoids is frequently prescribed for the following:

- Uncontrolled muscle spasms caused by multiple sclerosis and other degenerative diseases

- Nausea and vomiting among patients going through cancer chemotherapy

- Lack of appetite and weight loss caused by chronic illness, such as cancer and HIV

- Nerve pain

- Seizure disorders such as epilepsy

- Crohn's disease

Of course, if you are going to get Cannabis treatment, your doctor should be on board. Ideally, he or she should be the one to recommend the treatment for your specific condition. Once you and your doctor decide that you can benefit from Cannabis therapy, the next step is for you to acquire a "marijuana card" in those states with this practice. With this, you will be put on a list that permits you to buy medical marijuana from an authorized supplier that is called a dispensary.

All this is under the assumption that you reside in a state in the U.S. that has legalized medical marijuana. If you don't, then you will have to limit your options to FDA-approved medicines containing cannabinoids. Examples are Dronabinol and Nabilone, which are THC-containing medicines for the treatment of nausea and improvement of appetite. Another option is for you to use CBD Cannabis oil, which is legal in all parts of the U.S.

A third and more drastic option is to move to another state where medical marijuana is legal. Quite a number of people have been known to actually move residence precisely to be able to get legal marijuana treatment. Many of these are families with children suffering from epilepsy.

How Is Medical Marijuana Used?

The methods of marijuana treatment are identical to the ways by which weed is used recreationally. For instance, medical marijuana may be smoked by the patient. It too may be vaporized; in this method, the active ingredients are released through heating, without forming any smoke. Additionally, medical marijuana may also be ingested orally, or taken as tea, juice, or in a liquid extract form. Let's examine these methods more closely below.

Smoking Medical Cannabis

A popular way of taking medical marijuana is by smoking it in a pipe or joint. Through this method, the cannabinoid components (chiefly CBD and THC) are instantly absorbed into the lungs, then into the bloodstream, and finally across the blood-brain barrier. The effects of marijuana can therefore be felt within a few minutes. They dissipate more gradually, often after two or three hours.

Given this, smoked marijuana is very effective for treating acute symptoms that need immediate attention. Examples of these are acute pain, spasms, nausea and vomiting. It is also advantageous in that the patient can judge easily if he has taken enough and should stop. If the symptoms vanish, he can cease smoking. If they don't, he can continue smoking until he finds relief. (The process of measuring the correct amount to use is called *titrating*. To self-titrate means to gauge by yourself through experience how much you need.)

A disadvantage to smoked marijuana is that harmful substances in the smoke could irritate the lungs.

Vaporizing

This method is comparable to smoking, but a vape pen or a similar device is used instead. No smoke is produced because the marijuana is heated and not burned. Through heating, the active ingredients are released and then inhaled into the lungs. The effect is also instantaneously felt like in smoking. Doctors agree that vaporizing is as effective as, but healthier and more efficient than, smoking.

Ingesting Marijuana as Edibles

Cannabis edibles are food or snacks such as cookies, brownies, and candies. These are cooked using oil, butter, or ghee infused with marijuana. The effects of orally ingested Cannabis last longer than smoked or inhaled marijuana, usually between four to six hours after eating. However, the effects take longer to be felt, roughly 30 to 90 minutes after eating. This slow start and longer duration make Cannabis edibles the ideal method for treating chronic conditions that require a steady, continuous dose throughout the day.

Its disadvantage is the risk for overconsumption. It is difficult for the person to judge if he has eaten enough because the effects are slow to manifest. It is therefore recommended that he should generally eat a small amount, and then wait for about an hour before deciding if he needs to eat more.

This method is also not likely to be effective for the treatment of nausea, vomiting, and loss of appetite.

Drinking Cannabis Teas and Juices

Herbal Cannabis tea contains the raw, acidic, and non-psychoactive forms of THC and CBD which are named THCA and CBDA, respectively. These raw forms are not transformed into THC and CBD because steeping the tea does not provide a temperature that is high enough for decarboxylation to occur. (Decarboxylation refers to the process of applying heat to THCA and CBDA to transform them into THC and CBD, respectively.)

THCA and CBDA may not be as potent as THC and CBD, but they do appear to have medicinal properties. It is generally believed therefore that Cannabis tea may not be as effective or potent as other forms of the drug, but more research needs to be done to validate this opinion.

The same is true for Cannabis juice, as this also contains CBDA and THCA instead of CBD and THC.

It is harder to self-titrate when drinking herbal Cannabis tea or juice, but anecdotal evidence points it to be an effective and very easy way to get treatment.

Using Tinctures

Cannabis tinctures, common examples of which are green dragon and golden dragon, are made by dissolving marijuana in alcohol or a similar solvent. A small amount is then placed under the tongue, and you wait for it to work. Typically, 1 ml is recommended for first-time users. This often works adequately, but it can be increased to 2 ml the next day if the person feels a greater amount is needed.

The onset and duration of the effect of Cannabis tinctures is similar to that of edible Cannabis.

Using Sublingual Sprays

Sublingual sprays consist of cannabis extracts often mixed with another substance such as coconut oil. They are a concentrated form of marijuana that is sprayed under the tongue (that is, sublingually). The effects are quickly felt, generally within five to 15 minutes. This method is therefore well suited to the treatment of acute pain, as well as for medical conditions that require consistent and timely dosing. It is a quick, discreet, and smokeless (hence odorless) method preferred by many medical users of marijuana.

Using Cannabis Capsules and Gel Caps

Capsules and gel caps containing cannabis oil present another very easy method of treatment with medical marijuana. The patient simply takes the capsule in the same manner that he would drink any pill or multivitamin supplement. The dosing, effect, and duration are similar to that when ingesting edible Cannabis.

Using Topical Lotions and Salves

In this method, Cannabis oil and tinctures are infused in an ointment, lotion, or balm, and then rubbed on the skin. Alternatively, the oil or tincture is directly applied on the skin, without the need for it to be in lotion or ointment form. This method is suitable for treating skin conditions, pain, infections, and inflammation. It carries no risk of making you high.

Using Cannabis Oil Extracts

These oil extracts are made of concentrated marijuana, and as such are very potent. Many of them are CBD-rich and THC-dominant, and can therefore produce feelings of inebriation if a high dose is taken.

The oil extracts can be taken through a variety of ways: orally, sublingually, or via topical (skin) application. Additionally, they may be used as ingredients for cooking or for vaporizing. The onset and duration of effect differ, depending on how the oil extract is administered.

Medical Marijuana Side Effects

Some minor side effects may be experienced by those using Cannabis therapy. Thankfully, these side effects aren't very intense and they do not last long, if titration is done properly.

The side effects can include dizziness, sleepiness, short-term memory loss, and euphoric feelings or a high. In some cases, there are more serious side effects of psychosis and severe anxiety.

It is important to realize that these side effects depend not just on the dosage and Cannabis strain taken, but also on the sensitivity of the particular person to the drug. Medical marijuana is all about personalizing the drug to the specific disease and the unique characteristics of the individual user. There is no universal or "one size fits all" prescription for everyone.

It is thus imperative that the user properly consults with his doctor before proceeding with Cannabis therapy. This helps to ensure that the proper dosage and the correct drug ratio (of CBD to THC) are taken, so that unwanted side effects are avoided or kept to a minimum.

As an added precaution, a person should also refrain from taking medical marijuana if he or she:

- Has a heart condition

- Is pregnant

- Has a history of psychosis

- Is under 18 years old

6 MIRACLE CURES

Because of the great potential of marijuana — particularly its chief cannabinoids CBD and THC — as an effective cure for various medical conditions, a lot of research and development projects have focused on how it can be utilized most effectively and safely. The 1990s in particular were years that saw a huge upsurge in the number of clinical trials aimed at finding strains of marijuana that were most potent and at the same time had the least amount of undesirable side effects.

The focus of many of these medical studies was to develop safer, CBD-rich strains. A lot of work had to be done because for many years prior to the 1990s, the Cannabis industry in the United States had placed greater value on developing strains that had maximum THC to cater to recreational users. This was the case in Northern California, which was identified then as the country's "cannabis breadbasket."

Some of the notable companies and groups involved in this research were the Society of Cannabis Clinicians, the International Association for Cannabinoid Medicine (ICRS), Patients Out of Time, plus a good number of smaller clinics, laboratories, and research centers in the so-called "marijuana states," where medicinal marijuana was eventually legalized.

Pharmaceutical companies were not the only ones doing massive research into the potentials of medical Cannabis. Individuals — especially those who were personally invested in finding a cure for a disease that conventional medicine couldn't treat — also experimented with Cannabis oil. One such person was Rick Simpson. His name is famous in the CBD and marijuana industry, and you will understand why in the next section.

Rick Simpson: The Man Who Cured Cancer with Cannabis Oil

Rick Simpson was an ordinary Canadian who had an unfortunate accident in 1997 while he was working as an engineer in a hospital. He came in contact with asbestos in a poorly ventilated room, and inadvertently inhaled some of the noxious fumes. This caused him to pass out, and he was later taken to the hospital. Over the next days and weeks, he suffered from dizziness, headaches, terrible tinnitus (ringing in the ears), and generally feeling out of sorts. The tinnitus was very bad; Rick described it as like having a lawnmower right next to him. He was given medications, but they didn't help much.

A few years later, in 2003, he was diagnosed with a skin cancer called basal cell carcinoma. The doctors said it probably began with his asbestos accident. By this time, Rick was frustrated with the inability of his doctors and the medicines they were prescribing. He had suffered through a few years of poor health, and now he had cancer.

He remembered having heard about Cannabis earlier and how it could potentially help his case. He had expressed interest in the treatment before, prior to his cancer diagnosis, but this was brushed aside by his doctor. At that time, medicinal marijuana was practically unheard of. Nobody took it seriously. Now, with a confirmed cancer, Rick thought he had nothing to lose by trying out the unconventional treatment. In fact, he didn't seem to have any other choice given that his current treatment wasn't working.

We must remember that Rick didn't have any medical training. He certainly wasn't a doctor, and his own doctor didn't approve of him trying out Cannabis. But as mentioned, Rick felt that he had nothing to lose by experimenting with marijuana to treat his worsening condition.

And so, on his own, he found sources of cannabis and made oil out of it. He put this oil directly on his skin and on bandages that he also applied on himself. He got results just a few days afterwards. The alarming lumps on his arms and face immediately disappeared. His troubling tinnitus lessened and eventually was gone for good. For Rick, this was confirmation that cannabis oil could work miracles. It could cure cancer and he was living proof of it.

This was the start of Rick's career as a marijuana healer and activist. He went on to treat other people with cancer and skin diseases like himself. Most of them were patients who found no relief from conventional treatment programs in hospitals. They were people who had lost hope in modern medicine as they knew it. But with what came to be known later as the Rick Simpson Oil (RSO), their cancer and various ailments were cured. It was like a miracle.

Rick was eager to share his knowledge and his oil with everyone, especially those who needed it most. He helped treat thousands of patients — most, if not all of them — free of charge. These were not just people who had cancer, but included those who suffered from arthritis, diabetes, leukemia, AIDS or HIV, depression, insomnia, asthma, Crohn's disease, migraines, multiple sclerosis, and a host of other ailments. The simple secret, according to Rick, was to simply put Cannabis oil on the skin. In more serious medical conditions, the oil was ingested. Rick didn't espouse smoking or vaping as the mode of treatment using his cure.

Rick also became an influential campaigner for medical marijuana. He gave speeches, talked on the radio, travelled extensively to lecture, and wrote books on the therapeutic miracle of marijuana oil. He soon became a household name. His fame continued to rise as he carried on with his altruistic activities and his information campaigns about the effectiveness of Cannabis in general and RSO in particular.

How Cannabis Oil Worked to Cure Cancer

The interesting question to be addressed is how did Rick Simpson's Cannabis oil cure cancer? What was in it that successfully treated a dreaded disease that many other medicines couldn't cure? Without going into too much technicality, here are the salient points to know in order to answer that question:

- Cancer cells are actually produced in the human body continuously, but normally, our immune system destroys them before they can multiply too much. It is when our immune system is weak or compromised that cancerous growth intensifies unchecked and becomes a serious problem. This points out that, inherently, our body has the mechanism to fight and cure cancer.

- Within every cell are chemicals called *sphingolipids*. These dictate whether a cell will live or die. They also control the production of another chemical called *ceramides*, which in effect "kill" the cell after the decision that it will die has been made (by the sphingolipids). And so, if a cell has only a small number of ceramides, it is healthy and not dying any time soon. But if a cell has a high number of ceramides, it is nearing its death or destruction.

- When a cell becomes cancerous, its production of cannabinoid receptors increases. The higher number of these receptors alerts a part of our immune system called the endocannabinoid system to increase the production of ceramides.

- The ceramides produced then proceed to attack the mitochondria, which is the energy source of the cell. With a weakened mitochondria, the cell dies.

The essential takeaway from all this is simply that cannabinoids help to boost the immune system to fight cancer. Cannabinoids — which can be intrinsic in the body or taken from an external source like Cannabis oil — help to produce more ceramides that destroy the cancerous cells.

What is interesting is that this mechanism works not just with cancer cells, but with any other cell associated with infection or disease. This accounts for the versatility of cannabinoids (both THC and CBD) to cure various types of diseases.

That is a much simplified explanation for how Cannabis oil, or cannabinoids, work in fighting cancer and other diseases. If a more detailed explanation is needed, one would have to study the specific receptor sites on the cancer cells that are involved in this process, how the membranes on cellular mitochondria become more permeable to the action of certain destructive proteins, the ins and outs of what scientists call the "cancer cell death pathway," and so on.

What must be emphasized is that cannabinoids are highly effective because they very closely mimic the composition and action of natural chemicals in the body (the *endocannabinoids* mentioned before). If the immune system is weakened, as is the case when a person is sick, then introducing exocannabinoids (external cannabinoids such as those in Cannabis oil) into the body is perhaps the most natural and practical course of therapeutic action one can employ. It is a simple, non-aggressive yet highly effective mode of treatment that replicates how the body naturally combats diseases.

However, for effective Cannabis therapy, merely the infusion of cannabinoids into the body isn't enough. There must be a consistent and steady supply of these helpful chemicals, over a given period of time, for the treatment to be successful. This steady dosing ensures that ceramides continue to be produced and to accumulate, so that they can systematically and continuously destroy the cancerous or diseased cells, until these no longer pose a threat to the human system.

Other Medical Conditions that Cannabis Oil Is Most Effective For

Apart from cancer, medical marijuana has been demonstrated as most effective when used for the following:

- To treat severe pain. Marijuana can be used as a safer but also very potent alternative instead of narcotic painkillers.

- To ease the symptoms associated with a wide range of serious chronic conditions, such as HIV or AIDS, epilepsy, multiple sclerosis, Alzheimer's Disease, and Crohn's Disease

- To relieve nausea and other unpleasant side effects of chemotherapy treatment for cancer

- To stimulate appetite among patients with AIDS and other debilitating conditions

- To treat glaucoma

- To prevent or reduce muscle spasms in patients with neurological disorders

- As an adjunct medicine in the management of post-traumatic stress disease (PTSD) and other mental illnesses

For maximum efficacy, the use of marijuana should be supervised by a licensed physician. Needless to say, this can be done only in states where medical marijuana is legal. In states where it is not, the patient can opt to use CBD cannabis oil instead, as this is legal everywhere in the United States. Another alternative is to ask a doctor for FDA-approved medicines containing THC, an example of which is Marinol.

7 THE VARIOUS KINDS OF CANNABIS OIL

In many states in the U.S., the sale and use of medicinal marijuana is legally allowed. In others, it is not, though existing laws could change in the future to allow the legal use of Cannabis products to treat certain medical conditions.

The case with Cannabis oil, or CBD Cannabis oil to be exact, is slightly different. It is legal in all states, as long as it comes from industrial hemp. This condition ensures that the oil does not contain the psychoactive chemical that is THC. Thus, everyone in the United States can get their hands on CBD Cannabis oil, as it has become commercially available in the past few years, especially through online vendors.

If you're thinking of getting Cannabis oil, it would be a good idea to first know the main types: raw, decarboxylated, and filtered. I'll discuss these below.

Raw Cannabis Oil

This type contains CBD in addition to the chemicals that can ordinarily be found in hemp. It is therefore neither pure nor concentrated CBD oil, but is known to be effective for mild to moderate ailments. It is best used to relieve anxiety, sleeplessness or insomnia, stress, and depression. Generally, what it does is to promote a soothing effect.

Raw CBD oil is usually thick and has a dark green or blackish color. It is available in different strengths. It is the cheapest option among the three main types of Cannabis oil, because it has not been processed further after its extraction from the plant. Of the three, raw Cannabidoil also has the lowest percentage of CBD by volume. It is the type preferred by people who want the benefits of the entire Cannabis plant and not necessarily just the CBD component.

Decarboxylated Cannabis Oil

This is one step above raw Cannabis oil, in that it has been decarboxylated. The process of applying heat to decarboxylate the marijuana extract increases its strength, effectiveness and response time. It converts the acidic CBDA chemicals in the raw form to CBD, which is non-acidic and can therefore bind faster to natural CBD receptors in our body.

This type of oil is then more easily and more quickly processed once it is ingested into the body or rubbed on the skin.

Decarboxylated CBD oil is slightly more expensive than raw oil. It is available in different percentages of CBD content.

Filtered Cannabis Oil, or the "Gold" Line

This has the highest concentration of CBD among the cannabis oils. The raw form is carboxylated, and then filtered further to remove non-essential plant parts such as the lipids and chlorophyll. The resulting oil is golden in color, and is purer and thinner in consistency. It is more effective and faster-acting than the raw or decarboxylated variants. It also has a higher price tag, but this doesn't discourage buyers from choosing it over the others. Filtered gold Cannabis oil is the most popular and the most sought after of the three.

As a final note, it is worth mentioning that although these types are "oils," they are available in forms other than liquid oil. They can also be made into pastes, creams, ointments, suppositories, and capsules or pills — all of these are commercially sold for medical marijuana users.

8 LEGALITIES

First off, here's a quick background on early legislation concerning marijuana.

- Narcotics laws originally prohibited the use and selling of all marijuana extracts, and this covered even the non-psychoactive CBD-dominant strains.

- The first anti-marijuana law was passed in 1915 in the state of Utah, making it illegal to use Cannabis and its derivatives. After Utah, many other states followed suit and declared marijuana as a dangerous drug or controlled substance.

- In 1937, the U.S. Congress passed the Marihuana Tax Act, effectively prohibiting marijuana use all over the country.

- Decades later, in 1971, President Richard Nixon launched a "war on drugs" that further tightened the restrictions on Cannabis use. Marijuana was placed alongside harder drugs in the "most restricted" category.

- In the 1980s, President Ronald Reagan intensified the government's anti-drugs efforts, leading to unprecedented numbers of arrests and incarceration for marijuana use.

Afterwards, a reverse trend started. By the 1990s, much more had been learned (or re-discovered and brought out in the open) about Cannabis, particularly its medicinal value and its ability to treat ailments that conventional medicines cannot cure. People who experienced first-hand the therapeutic miracles of the plant talked about it, activists like Rick Simpson began campaigning for its legalization, and the movement to lift the ban against marijuana was born. The government (or at least certain states) listened and capitulated to what the public wanted, in the face of undeniable evidence that marijuana has great medicinal value that far outweighs the risks.

A landmark event was the legalization of medical marijuana in 1996 in the state of California with the passing of Proposition 215. In the same year, the first marijuana dispensary, called Marin Alliance, opened in Fairfax, California. Soon after, other states also legalized medical marijuana. These were Oregon (in 1998, through the Oregon Medical Marijuana Act), Maine (1999), Nevada and Colorado (2000), Montana (2004), Vermont and New Mexico (2007), Michigan (2008), Arizona and New Jersey (2010), Massachusetts (2012), and Minnesota and New York (2014). In 2016, Ohio and Pennsylvania legalized medical marijuana through legislature, and Florida, North Dakota, and Arkansas also legalized medical Cannabis via ballot initiative. To date, 19 states have legalized marijuana, and this number could increase in the coming years.

The legal status of cannabis in the state of Utah is slightly different and rather interesting for those of us who are studying CBD Cannabis oil. Utah has not legalized medical marijuana, but it legalized CBD oil in 2014. Similarly, Oklahoma also legalized trials of CBD oil in the same year (2014). Two other states, namely Georgia and Texas, later also legalized CBD oil, in 2015.

Thus, apart from the nineteen states where medical marijuana is now legal, four additional states have legalized CBD Cannabis oil, bringing the total to 23 states.

Other important laws and legislation worth noting are the following:

- In 2008, Massachusetts decriminalized cannabis.

- In 2012, Washington and Colorado legalized the recreational use of marijuana for adults (those 21 years old or older).

- In 2014, Maryland followed suit, decriminalizing marijuana.

- In 2014, Alaska and Oregon also legalized recreational marijuana, with the effectivity dates starting in February 2015 (for Alaska) and July 2015 (for Oregon).

- In 2015 and 2016, cannabis was also decriminalized in Delaware, Illinois, California, Nevada, Maine, and Massachusetts

The Legal Status of CBD Cannabis Oil

Backing up a bit, I want to reiterate here an important point that was mentioned in an earlier section: that CBD-rich low-THC marijuana oil, or Cannabis oil, is legal in *all* states, under the assumption that it is derived from industrial hemp. This condition ensures that the Cannabis oil does not contain THC, or any amount of THC that could produce a psychoactive effect in the person who takes or uses the oil.

Legal marijuana oil or Cannabis oil is very much like hemp oil and hempseed oil, which are considered to be dietary supplements and not technically medicine. These oils, as discussed earlier, have virtually zero THC content, and therefore do not cause any hallucinogenic effects.

The main point that it is impossible to get high from cannabidiol derived from industrial hemp. Thus, it is legal to purchase and consume wherever you are in the United States. CBD hemp oil is also legal in more than 40 other countries besides the United States. These include Mexico, Brazil, Canada, France, and China.

Now here's another fine detail that we must be aware of. It is legal in the United States to use CBD Cannabis oil, but it is *not* legal to cultivate hemp or marijuana, even if the intention is to produce industrial hemp. In other words, the planting or growing of marijuana is illegal, generally speaking. The reason for this is that while growers use mostly the stems and roots to make fiber or oil, there is nothing to stop them from using the flowers and leaves to produce recreational marijuana or weed. In other words, it is a liability to have the *whole* marijuana plant, even if the intention is to just use the stems and roots.

As such, most hemp oil is imported from countries outside the United

States. It isn't available locally because of the legal restriction against the cultivation of the hemp plant. A few companies are able to legally grow Cannabis in the country, but they had to pass through a very stringent process before they were allowed to do so. The government imposes very strict conditions before giving anyone the permission to grow hemp. In consequence, most companies just don't bother to go through the process; instead, they just import hemp because this is so much easier to do.

Other Pertinent Laws and Restrictions Concerning Marijuana

Regardless of where you live in the United States, the following laws on marijuana apply:

- Marijuana and its extracts are illegal to transport across state lines. But CBD Cannabis oil is not covered by this restriction.

- It is always illegal to drive when stoned.

- It is illegal to use marijuana if the person is younger than 21 years, unless he or she is a medical marijuana patient.

These and similar laws should not be taken lightly, as they are implemented strictly by the authorities. In spite of the law reforms in different states, we still see incredibly huge numbers of arrests related to marijuana use or possession on a yearly basis. These arrests outnumber the combined total arrests for all cruel crimes. To cite an example, in 2014, close to three-quarters of a million people were arrested for marijuana violations. This number corresponds to almost half (45 percent) of all drug arrests in the country. It is also equivalent to roughly 1 arrest every 50 seconds, something that just boggles the mind.

9 SUMMARY AND FINAL WORDS

The main theme of this book is the enormous medicinal benefits that can be derived from the Cannabis plant and its extracts. But Cannabis use can cause intoxication and other forms of short-term mental impairment. If the purpose of using marijuana is medicinal, this is an unwanted side effect. To avoid it, the best thing to do is to take CBD-dominant marijuana. This doesn't contain the chemical THC, which is the cannabinoid responsible for the hallucinogenic effects of marijuana. CBD-dominant Cannabis is commercially available as CBD cannabis oil, and is legal to use in all states in the country.

Another main idea presented in this book is that marijuana has long been used as a recreational drug and as an effective all-around cure for numerous medical conditions. Its use dates back to prehistoric times and continues up to the present. The most common medicinal uses of marijuana are:

- To relieve all kinds of pain, including headaches, muscle pain, neuralgia, and menstrual cramps

- To relieve inflammation

- To ease the symptoms of debilitating chronic diseases such as cancer, Alzheimer's disease, epilepsy, rheumatism, Crohn's disease, diabetes, and many others

- To alleviate the nausea and vomiting that usually accompanies chemotherapy

- To stimulate appetite and encourage weight gain among patients with chronic illnesses

- To calm anxiety, relieve stress, and lessen other symptoms of mental illness

Marijuana oil has even been used to treat serious conditions like cancer. The experience of Rick Simpson and his Cannabis oil bears this out.

Medical marijuana has been legalized in more than 20 states in the U.S., and this number could increase in the coming years. And as mentioned, CBD-dominant marijuana oil is legal all over the country. Given these, it is possible for anyone to take advantage of the incredible health and medical benefits that the marijuana plant offers.

CONCLUSION

Thank you for taking the time to read this book.

You should now have a good understanding of medical marijuana as well as cannabidiol (CBD) — and its uses for wellness.

If you enjoyed this book, please take the time to leave me a review on Amazon. I appreciate your honest feedback, and it really helps me to continue producing high-quality books.

Simply go here to leave a review: https://www.amazon.com/dp/B01NBUX8VZ#customerReviews

And please join my mailing list. You can go here to sign up: https://joannehillyerwrites.wixsite.com/home. You can look forward to bonus content, reader surveys, and announcements about upcoming books.

ABOUT THE AUTHOR

Joanne Hillyer has a lifelong interest in wellness, healthy eating, alternative medicine, and the outdoors. She is especially interested in using easily found tools and ingredients for improving healthy living. Born and raised in the Pacific Northwest, she enjoys the great outdoors, travel, cooking, and walking.

Made in the USA
Columbia, SC
19 December 2018